Summary of

Being Mortal

by Atul Gawande

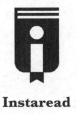

Instaread

Please Note

This is key takeaways and analysis.

Table of Contents

Overview

Being Mortal, written by Atul Gawande, brings to light an array of concepts involving death, mortality, aging, and terminal illness. Gawande includes extensive research and chronicles the stories of his patients, other doctors' patients, and his own family members. The resulting book informs readers about many circumstances and scenarios that can help people find the best route through their or their family members' final days, months, or years.

Gawande runs through the history and practicality of common ways the sick and elderly live when taking care of themselves becomes unmanageable. These primarily include hospitals, nursing homes, assisted living, and hospice. He examines the positives and negatives of each while discussing the spectrum of autonomy each option allows. Autonomy is an important concept both to Gawande's narrative and anyone who faces sickness, aging, and death. Gawande explores other concepts and scenarios faced by the dying, such as whether to pursue treatment to the end, despite the fact that those treatments could sacrifice quality of life or shorten life.

Interspersed throughout the book are personal stories weaved in and out of Gawande's research, conceptual explanations, and analysis. These stories illustrate many of the different points he makes. Included is a detailed account of the end of his father's life and his father's struggle to maintain a life he could enjoy while battling a paralyzing tumor. Gawande calls for doctors to examine their pursuits with their own patients who face imminent death, and stresses the importance of palliative care going forward.

Important People

Atul Gawande: Gawande is the author of the book, but he also played a role, either as a doctor or a relative, in some of the personal stories he shares throughout the book.

Atmaram Gawande: Atmaram was Gawande's father. He was diagnosed with a tumor in his spinal cord. Gawande chronicles his life from pre-tumor through death in the book.

Alice Hobson: Alice was the grandmother of Gawande's wife. She represented one of Gawande's first encounters with aging and mortality.

Sitaram Gawande: Sitaram was Gawande's grandfather in India who lived independently to an old age while being cared for by many members of his family. In the book, Gawande uses Sitaram as an example of the old way of taking care of the elderly before modern medicine.

Lou Sanders: Lou was an elderly man who moved in with his daughter as he grew older. He later struggled in an assisted living home when caring for him became too much for the daughter.

Sara Monopoli: Sara was only in her thirties and pregnant with her first child when she found out she was going to die of lung cancer. Gawande uses her story as an example of how continuing treatments against all odds is not always the best healthcare strategy.

Peg Bachelder: Peg was the piano teacher of Gawande's daughter, Hunter. She had a rare, soft-tissue cancer and eventually went on hospice, but she continued giving piano lessons until the end of her life because it gave her purpose.

Key Takeaways

1. Nursing homes were not created to assist the elderly with their dependency on others or provide a better option than poorhouses. They were created to clear out hospital beds.

2. Assisted living arose from the need for an alternative to nursing homes that could give patients more independence and control over their lives.

3. At the end of their lives, most people want more than to merely survive, which is where medical institutions, nursing homes, and assisted living can fall flat.

4. People need to ask themselves what would make life worth living when they are ill, old, frail, or dependent on others for daily care.

5. People who have the end of life discussion can alleviate the burden and confusion felt by themselves, their families, and their doctors when death is eminent, and it can contribute to a better quality of life.

6. When facing death, people need to determine how far they are willing to go with treatment to extend life that could, ultimately, come at the cost of their quality of life.

7. Nursing homes and assisted living are often devised more for the benefit of patients' children

rather than patients themselves, and the children are often the decision makers for patients at the end of their lives.

8. Autonomy is a crucial human need that is often forgotten or ignored as people near death.

9. Hospice care does not mean surrendering to death, but can instead be a way for patients to improve their quality of life.

10. Doctors often struggle with speaking to their patients about the realities of their health and the potential outcomes of treatment.

11. Doctors and society have the opportunity to alter the perception of illness, aging, and death. With this change in perception, they can transform the institutions, culture, and conversations to ultimately improve the end of people's lives.

Thank you for purchasing this Instaread book

**Download the Instaread mobile app to get
unlimited text & audio summaries
of bestselling books.**

Visit Instaread.co
to learn more.

Analysis

Key Takeaway 1

Nursing homes were not created to assist the elderly with their dependency on others or provide a better option than poorhouses. They were created to clear out hospital beds.

Analysis

In the industrialized world, hospitals transformed the way people looked at illness, aging, and death. Hospitals became the norm for people with bodily ailments, including those caused by aging, and hospitals soon filled to capacity with sick and elderly people with nowhere else to go. To alleviate this problem, the government funded separate units that hospitals created to tend to those needing extended recovery. Hospitals began clearing out beds and funneling those patients into what became known as nursing homes.

The initial intention of nursing homes was not directly related to improving care for the terminally ill and the elderly, thus nursing homes often did not meet the expectations of the patients or their families. Though some consider it a problem of the past, many nursing homes still do not operate in the better interest of its patients' quality of life. Health and safety remain paramount, but that is often at the expense of patients' happiness and sense of fulfillment in life.

When caring for a number of ill and otherwise dependent people in one place, caregivers fall back on schedules for everything from eating and taking medications to activities and socializing. Rigid schedules negate one of the fundamental needs of humans. This need is the feeling that they can do what they want, when they want, which is stripped away by the common management strategies of nursing homes.

This is not necessarily the fault of an individual nursing home, but rather the fundamental purpose of nursing homes as an institution. Gawande notes one sociologist compares nursing homes to prisons, military training camps, orphanages, and mental hospitals, all of which he calls total institutions. A total institution does away with the barriers separating the spheres of life, such as sleeping, working, and playing, and funnels them into one place and schedule. The institutionalization of the dying process devalues the quality and purpose of life in the final days, months, or years.

Key Takeaway 2

Assisted living arose from the need for an alternative to nursing homes that could give patients more independence and control over their lives.

Analysis

Assisted living offers patients more autonomy that nursing homes took away once a patient entered the facility. With its rigid schedules and limited grounds, nursing homes, by design, control residents' lives to ensure their health and safety above all else. While these are noble and fundamental causes, most people still want to be able to control their decision making and what happens to them on a day to day basis.

Even if residents are physically limited, they desire some semblance of independence and control, and assisted living provides those opportunities more so than nursing homes. While nursing homes do have the word home in their name, they are not actual homes, and residents might not consider them homes while residing there.

Assisted living facilities, on the other hand, offer residents a place they could call home. In their own home, they set the ground rules. They decide what possessions they can have and where to place them. They decide who can enter and when they can lock their own doors. With assisted living, residents' priorities take precedence over the priorities of management and caretakers that govern nursing homes.

However, where nursing homes and assisted living do agree is that their residents do still need a certain amount of attention from caretakers. With both assisted living and nursing homes, residents have access to nurses to help them with medical care, often twenty-four hours a day. They also often have someone to help them take care of basic needs, such as personal hygiene or chores around the home, if needed.

Key Takeaway 3

At the end of their lives, most people want more than to merely survive, which is where medical institutions, nursing homes, and assisted living can fall flat.

Analysis

At the core of human needs are survival and safety, as they have been for thousands of years. When it comes to medicine and end of life care, these two needs remain paramount above all else, and they shape the way people and doctors have come to see the dying process.

As civilization developed, other needs came into focus, such as emotions, self-worth, fulfillment, purpose, loyalty, and independence. In modern day society, these needs are at the forefront of most people's minds over merely safety and survival. At the end of life, those needs do not change. They have become as fundamental to quality of life as the simple need to maintain life.

These needs and overall quality of life often fall by the wayside when it comes time for end-of-life care. This can come at a cost to a dying person's health, both mentally and physically. Gawande explores several needs humans continue to seek even to the end. One is finding a cause beyond themselves, such as living for family or to take care of a pet or project. He describes this as loyalty, the opposite of individualism. People want to be a part of something greater to transcend to a level of self-actualization where they can enable others to achieve their own potential.

Nursing homes and assisted living do not always attend to these needs. In caring for an aging or dying person, caregivers only focus on physical care rather than providing or encouraging opportunities to help patients seek fulfillment in their lives.

Key Takeaway 4

People need to ask themselves what would make life worth living when they are ill, old, frail, or dependent on others for daily care.

Analysis

Gawande questions why simple existence, or being housed, fed, safe, and alive, produces a life that feels empty and meaningless to many people. People must determine the answer as to what would make their lives be worth living when they become ill, old, or otherwise dependent on others, thus losing some control over their daily lives. To ascribe meaning to life is different for every individual with their own experiences, hopes, dreams, pleasures, and desires. This meaning could be anything from keeping in contact with family members to being able to eat the foods they enjoy.

Figuring out what makes life worth living is a crucial part of being able to ensure a quality of life when people reach the end of their lives. Many people, however, either do not determine what they want, or they wait until it is too late to communicate and carry out the plan. Aging, illness, and accidents can lead to an inability to communicate, think clearly, or participate in activities they love, so people need to figure out these wants out sooner than later. Before the worst happens, determining wants and communicating them with family and doctors can lead to a more fulfilling and meaningful life at the end of the road.

Key Takeaway 5

People who have the end of life discussion can alleviate the burden and confusion felt by themselves, their families, and their doctors when death is eminent, and it can contribute to a better quality of life.

Analysis

After deciding how they want to spend the the end of their life, people must have this important discussion with those on whom they depend to be responsible for actualizing those wants. Many people avoid this conversation, deeming it negative and defeatist. While it may be difficult in the moment, what they do not realize is that having this discussion can actually greatly improve their quality of life and possibly even help them live longer lives.

Gawande cites research confirming that many do not have this discussion with their families and doctors, but the ones who do often need less critical medical care, enroll in hospice, suffer less, are more physically capable, and could interact with others better and for a longer time. Research also found that families who had this discussion showed signs of depression for less time following the death of their loved one.

Dying at peace is important to many people, and if more of them realized how important having the end of life discussion is, quality of life for the dying in general could greatly improve. In turn, healthcare costs for families, providers, and the government may decrease. Sometimes the patient cannot initiate the conversation themselves. It is then up to the family and doctors to encourage the discussion so that they can utilize the best system of care and ensure the patient's happiness as they approach death.

Key Takeaway 6

When facing death, people need to determine how far they are willing to go with treatment to extend life that could, ultimately, come at the cost of their quality of life.

Analysis

A crucial part of the end of life discussion is how much treatment the patient is willing to endure to extend the amount of time they have. The discussion also needs to cover what quality of life the patient is willing to sacrifice along the way. Oftentimes when patients near death, particularly with a terminal illness, doctors can offer any number of possible treatments that could sustain life for a little longer. This may be enticing to patients and their families. While they are available, these treatments do not always promise much, if any, additional time that a patient can live, and they certainly do not focus on the patient's quality of life.

Sometimes, additional treatments can put patients through great amounts of pain and anguish just to secure a few more days, weeks, or months of life. Still worse, sometimes these treatments can actually worsen a patient's condition or even result in death. To take such risks to have a little more time together is not always worth going through for patients or for their families.

People must face this question and find the answer for themselves. They should determine how many, if any, chemotherapy treatments they would be willing to undergo to treat a cancerous tumor, or what type of surgery they would agree to, no matter the risks or results. They need to figure out if the doctors should try to resuscitate them, even if that means sustaining life only on feeding tubes and artificial life support. Sometimes people consider these medical interventions a loss of dignity, but others are willing to try anything to keep on living. People need to think about the quality of life they want in the end and what they are willing to suffer through before either dying or choosing hospice care.

Key Takeaway 7

Nursing homes and assisted living are often devised more for the benefit of patients' children rather than patients themselves, and the children are often the decision makers for patients at the end of their lives.

Analysis

According to Gawande, many people believe that assisted living developed more as a way to appease a patient's children rather than the patient themselves. At the end of life, many people surrender their decision making to their children as they may not always be in the proper state of mind to make such decisions themselves.

As a result, assisted living facilities often tend to sell themselves to a patient's children instead of the patient. This is usually with a certain look, a list of amenities, and activities that children believe their parents would like. While the children may mean well in selecting a facility they believe is best for their parent, they do not always ask or consider the parent and what their needs or desires are. This can result in a satisfied child but a very unsatisfied parent, the person who must actually live their days in the facility.

The facility may offer a variety of amenities and activities, but they may not be tailored toward the interests of a particular patient. The facility may offer an around the clock nursing staff, but the patient may want more independence in how and when they receive visits or take their medications. Any number of reasons can turn off a patient to a certain facility that, to the child, seems like a perfect fit. Children need to try to see a facility not with their own wants in mind, but with the needs and desires of the parent who will live there.

Key Takeaway 8

Autonomy is a crucial human need that is often forgotten or ignored as people near death.

Analysis

As society has evolved, so too has the veneration of certain ideals. For a long time, particularly before modern medicine, people aspired to simply grow older. As medicine progressed and more people began living to see an older age, this aspiration changed. Instead of aspiring to be young, however, people now aspire to be, and remain, independent or autonomous.

Autonomy is one of the most critical needs that people of all ages strive to maintain, but autonomy begins to slip away as illness and the aging process give way to more dependence on others. However, to many people who founded facilities to care for the elderly, they believe that people do not have to sacrifice their autonomy just because they are becoming more dependent.

Gawande describes two forms of autonomy. The first is for people to have complete freedom and control over their day to day lives, and the second is the ability to remain the author of their own life's story. As they age, people may no longer be able to drive themselves to the grocery store or dress themselves in the morning. That dependence, however, should not negate the fact that those people have the desire to have more groceries in their home or want to be more presentable as their day begins. While actions themselves may become dependent on others for help, the desires and motivations behind those actions should remain in the hands and minds of the sick and elderly.

Families and caregivers may easily forget the importance of a person's autonomy, particularly as they near death. It could come at great cost to the person's quality of life and even overall mental and physical health. Autonomy is not just a desire, not something that is nice to have, but rather an intrinsic human need, even until the end of people's lives.

Key Takeaway 9

Hospice care does not mean surrendering to death, but can instead be a way for patients to improve their quality of life.

Analysis

Sometimes, people equate hospice to giving up on life and surrendering to illness. Indeed, the decision to choose hospice care can be a strange and difficult choice for patients, as they choose to face death and a better quality of life rather than face treatments and the potential to live longer.

Gawande illustrates the difference between standard medical care and hospice, which mainly comes down to priorities. Medical care focuses on the future and keeping someone alive to see that future, sometimes regardless of how extending life can sacrifice quality of life. On the other hand, hospice focuses on helping a patient live a full life in that moment without as much emphasis on when, exactly, death will come.

What is crucial to understand about hospice, however, is not just the nature of care present at the end of life. This type of care can actually contribute to extending life as well. When people stop fighting against aging and sickness with potentially risky and damaging treatments, they could be avoiding the treatments that might ultimately bring them to death more quickly. In short, choosing hospice over treatment can actually be a form of choosing life.

As incomes rise and people become more focused on quality of life rather than simply living, hospice is becoming a more common way for people to spend the end of their lives. Whether that be a few days before death spent with family surrounding them, or a few months of at least partial independence and control over their lives, people are seeing and appreciating the value of hospice over risky treatments.

Key Takeaway 10

Doctors often struggle with speaking to their patients about the realities of their health and the potential outcomes of treatment.

Analysis

According to Gawande, when it comes to illness, aging, and death, doctors do not always approach the conversations they need to have with their patients in the best way. They often focus on facts and figures and do not always release full information about a patient's true prognosis. They may offer treatments they know have a slim chance of success. When they take a more paternalistic role, doctors may try to control a situation and offer what they think is best for the patient rather than being informative or even collaborative in determining the best route for care.

While doctors may feel they are protecting their patients, they are actually performing a great disservice. Doctors sometimes give patients false hope about the true efficacy of a particular treatment or overestimate to patients how long they will live. In doing so, doctors may be discouraging or preventing their patients from having the discussions and making the decisions they need as death approaches. If patients think they have a chance to live longer, they may not face the reality and nearness of death. It is the doctor's ultimate responsibility to adjust their patients' expectations to be more realistic and productive.

Doctors also need to focus less on the science of a diagnosis and treatment. They should focus more on the impact that news can have on patients. Doctors need to be able to temper anxiety through comforting words and actions rather than just providing a stoic overview of facts and the biological processes involved. Patients depend on their doctors for both information and a sense of stability when dealing with highly emotional and sometimes painful news. More doctors should take it upon themselves to be as valuable to their patients as possible.

Key Takeaway 11

Doctors and society have the opportunity to alter the perception of illness, aging, and death. With this change in perception, they can transform the institutions, culture, and conversations to ultimately improve the end of people's lives.

Analysis

Through the course of history, the perception of what old age is and what it means has changed dramatically, particularly in the past century, thanks to modern medicine. Not only do people live longer, but as the baby boomer generation edges toward retirement age, the country's elderly population is stretching toward new heights. This means needing new strategies for taking care of a significantly older population.

More people in the U.S. are turning to hospice as a way to spend the end of their lives. This trend may continue into the coming decades and may possibly become the new norm for caring for the sick and elderly. The institutionalization of dying may either change drastically or come to pass as the country adopts new perceptions of the elderly and devises a new culture that surrounds them. Discussions for end of life care may not only increase but improve, which can in turn boost the quality of life for the elderly population as a whole.

The responsibility for this movement falls not only on society, but on doctors who play a role in how society sees the elderly. Instead of treating old age as a societal, non-medical issue, doctors can find new ways to not just treat the elderly's symptoms, but to alleviate their worries and improve their quality of life.

Author's Style

Gawande examines many concepts related to aging, terminal illness, and the dying process as well as how aging and dying individuals are treated within medical settings, families, and society as a whole. He does not misrepresent the facts or leave out the benefits and drawbacks of one side or the other. He does, however, interject his opinions about how the dying should be treated and what medicine, families, and society can do to improve their lives.

The book's chapters and sections are fairly long and packed with historical references, research, personal stories, and analysis. Each chapter has a simple, specific heading dealing with the end of life that then guides the amalgam of literary devices the author uses to illuminate each subject in detail.

Gawande chooses several different personal stories from his patients, other doctors' patients, and his own family to provide examples for different concepts he discusses. He bookends Being Mortal with personal stories, beginning with one of his first encounters with death, that of his future wife's grandmother, and ending with his most personal account, that of his father. Throughout the book, he continues to reference those two stories, but he also tells other stories of people who went down their own paths to death. He explores the history and realities of the stories while using them as avenues for a larger description of the dying process and how it affects the patients and their families.

In addition to telling the stories of patients and their families, Gawande also interviews figures who offer history and opinions of some of the concepts he explores. These include the founders of assisted living homes, caretakers, and other physicians and figures in the medical field.

Author's Perspective

As a successful surgeon, Gawande often narrates from the perspective of a doctor. He explains certain practices in medicine and relationships with patients. At other times, he laments the shortfalls of his fellow doctors and how the group as a whole can make the field of medicine a better place for the dying. Gawande also takes the position of the reader or common man who is curious and concerned about the path his or her own life will take when he or she is on the verge of death.

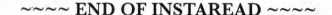

~~~~ END OF INSTAREAD ~~~~

Thank you for purchasing this Instaread book

**Download the Instaread mobile app to get
unlimited text & audio summaries
of bestselling books.**

Visit Instaread.co
to learn more.

CPSIA information can be obtained
at www.ICGtesting.com
Printed in the USA
LVOW13s1506300718
585374LV00017B/419/P